# Healthy Essential Oils Guide For Skin Care, Hair, Allergies, Weight Loss, Natural Cleaning

*47 NEW Essential Oils Recipes To Heal, Build And Improve Your Health For Beginners*

KATHY LEWIS

ISBN-10: 1522997741
ISBN-13: 978-1522997740

# CONTENTS

# Introduction

I want to thank and congratulate you for downloading this book « Healthy Essential Oils Guide For Skin Care, Hair, Allergies, Weight Loss, Natural Cleaning: 47 NEW Essential Oils Recipes To Heal, Build And Improve Your Health For Beginners».

If you're looking for balance, for beauty products based on plants and essential oils, if you long for a more serene and pure lifestyle, without turning your present habits and ways upside down, this little guide is for you. Circulatory problems, cellulite, flabby stomach, constipation, toxin elimination, stimulants or draining products, beauty masks...

This straightforward and practical guide contains my little recipes, all tested by me in my mountain chalet. All my friends agree: these recipes are effective, pleasant and economical. Why spend a fortune, when generous Nature is there, ready to provide all that you need?

In short, here is a gentle solution for your body-care, which you can prepare and use within your own four walls.

The little recipes below will bring you second-to-none bodily comfort and well-being. Adopt bio products for a healthy body. Learn to love yourself – take some time just for you. It's really important.

## The Definition of Natural Essential Oils

Essential oils contain the true essence of the plant they are derived from. The liquid essential oil is usually distilled by a steam or water process, from the flowers, leaves, stems, bark, roots, or other elements of a plant. You might be surprised to discover essential oils don't actually feel oily. Most essential oils are clear, except for a few oils like lemongrass, patchouli, or orange, which are yellow or amber in color.

Don't confuse therapeutic essential oils and fragrance oils, which aren't the same. Fragrance oils are perfume oils, containing synthetic chemicals, and they have absolutely no therapeutic value.
In the United States, there are no aromatherapy regulations or regulations on how the term aromatherapy is used. When buying commercial products, remember they could contain ingredients that use fragrance oil or synthetic chemicals. Carefully read all the ingredients.

Even when a manufacturer claims a product contains natural ingredients, or that they are made from essential oils, you must be careful. Even when the product says it is made only from natural ingredients, it can still contain fragrance oils or other synthetic products. Only a couple of drops of essential oil are needed to be able to claim a product is 'made with essential oils.

The best way to be sure that you have a high-quality therapeutic product is to make your own products, and we will provide you with some great recipes to get you started and help you to develop your skills. Before long, you will be a master at creating these recipes.
The quality and price of essential oil can vary significantly, depending on a number of factors, which include whether the botanical is rare, where it the botanical comes from, the conditions it is grown in, the standards of the distiller, and the amount of oil that can be produced.

## The Benefits of Applying Essential Oils to Your Skin

When you apply essential oils to your skin, they are directly absorbed into your bloodstream allowing you to enjoy the constituents of that particular essential oils and the health benefits associated with it. Essential oils are highly concentrated so most essential oils should never be applied directly to your skin without first diluting them using one of the common carrier oils like sweet almond oil – more on these a little later.

## The Benefits of Inhaling Essential Oils

When you inhale an essential oil, it can offer both mental and physical benefits. The aroma of the essential oil will stimulate your brain to trigger a specific reaction and when you inhale an essential oil into your lungs, the active chemicals will provide therapeutic benefits. For example, diffusing eucalyptus essential oil can relieve congestion from a cold.

It is extremely important that essential oils are always correctly and safely used so that you can enjoy the benefits without the negative consequences. Essential oils are medicinal, and you need to recognize them as such.

In addition to therapeutic benefits, essential oils can be used to make your own insect repellents, diffusers, beauty products, laundry cleaners, household products, and more.

## Essential Oil Blends

You can blend together two or more essential oils to create both intricate aromas and therapeutic blends. When essential oils are blended with a specific therapeutic function, they are called essential oil synergy. A synergistic essential oil blend's total action is significantly greater than when each essential oil is independently used.

## 9 Essential Oil Safety Guidelines

Essential oils are very concentrated. It is important that you understand essential oil safety, because when they are not correctly used they can be harmful. Bringing aromatherapy into your life should not cause you to worry, but you must treat therapeutic essential oils as medicines. These basic safety guidelines will ensure you safely enjoy the benefits of aromatherapy. You should not consider this a complete reference. Anytime you are unsure, talk to your doctor or an aromatherapy practitioner.

1. Some essential oils can cause allergic reactions or sensitization in a small number of people. Therefore, the first time you use an essential oil topically, you should do a skin patch test on a small area of skin.

2. Never use an essential oil undiluted on your skin. Occasionally an experienced user will make an exception to this precaution, but you should not do this until you have significant knowledge about essential oils. Until then never apply an essential oil to your skin until you have diluted it with a carrier oil.

3. Some essential oils are phototoxic. These essential oils can cause blistering, inflammation, redness, or burning when they are exposed to UVA rays.

4. If you have epilepsy, are pregnant, asthma, or a health condition, there are some essential oils that you should not use. Before using any essential oil, you need to do your research and review all safety precautions associated with each essential oil.

5. Less is better. When you use essential oils, you should use the smallest amount of essential oil that is effective For example, if 1-2 drops are called for, start with one drop and see how that goes, then up to two drops if one is ineffective. Essential oils are concentrated and using more is wasteful.

6. Not all essential oils should be used in aromatherapy. Onion, camphor, pennyroyal, wormwood, bitter almond, etc. are examples of a few of the essential oils that you should not use in aromatherapy.

7. Store essential oils away from kids. Some essential oils like citrus oils can smell good and your child might be tempted to drink them so store out of the reach of children. After all, they are medicines that are potentially poisonous in the hands of children.

8. Don't ingest essential oils. The only time you should ingest essential oils is when a qualified aromatherapy practitioner prescribes or you have a recipe that you completely trust.

9. Essential oils are flammable. Store essential oils away from fire hazards.

# 1 - Essential Oil Recipes Greasy, Dry, Acne Skin

### 1. Mask for Greasy Skin

I tested this recipe on a friend. It really helped reduce the oozing of her skin.

*Recipe:*

- Steep some rose petals in a little rosewater and glycerin
- Crush 3 large, ripe strawberries
- Add to these a soup-spoonful of flour and a whole egg

*Directions:*

1. Mix it all well and apply to your face, especially to the forehead, around the nostrils and on the chin.
2. Leave for ten minutes and then rinse off.

### 2. Beauty Masks for Dry Skin

Avocado oil is widely used in cosmetics. It tones and regenerates the skin. It makes an excellent anti-wrinkle mask or capillary mask prior to shampooing to stimulate a dry scalp (pour one teaspoonful onto the scalp and massage briskly, for a sort of scrubbing effect. Then shampoo and rinse well, finishing with a cold rinse which will close up the pores of your skin and tone the scalp.
Glowing result guaranteed).

*Recipe:*

- Crush the pulp of a very ripe avocado until it is creamy
- Add the juice of half a lemon
- Two soup-spoons full of fresh cream

## *Directions:*

1. Apply to face and neck.
2. Leave for ten minutes, then rinse away.

### 3. Acne Recipe

## *Recipe:*

- 2 oz. jojoba oil
- 8 drops lavender essential oil
- 10 drops tea tree essential oil

## *Directions:*

1. Pour the jojoba into a clean glass bottle.
2. Add the essential oils and seal the bottle then gently roll back and forth for a couple of minutes to ensure mix.
3. Apply a small amount to acne.

# 2 - Healthy Essential Oil Recipes For Abdomen Problems

### 4.  Essential Oil Mouthwash for Ulcers

*Recipe:*

- 2 drops of tea tree oil
- 2 drops of geranium oil
- 2 drops of thyme oil
- 2 drops of lemon oil
- 2 drops of peppermint oil
- 10 ml brandy

*Directions:*

1. Mix all the oils and dissolve a teaspoon in a glass of water, swish around your mouth then spit out.

### 5.  Cellulite Problems

You want to get rid of your cellulite, but the products available for sale are too expensive. You can make your own plasters, completely free, using natural ingredients.

*Recipe:*

- Strip the leaves from some ivy

- Reduce the ivy leaves to a pulp. You can find ivy all over the place, in woods but also growing on walls in town.
- Mix in a little grape seed oil and apply to the affected areas, massaging firmly.
- Leave for half an hour then rinse well with cool water!

This treatment, combined with palpation, will bring back your figure and wipe out your cellulite.

### Palpation to Slim Stomach:
To decongest fat layers, nothing is more effective than palpation.

### Manual Method:
Take a fold of skin between thumb and fingers, with both hands close together, and then roll the skin steadily backwards and forwards.

Although painful, this is very effective if done using an ivy-based plaster.

P.S.: A tip! avoid........

- Hard cheese, choose soft cheeses, rich in protein (8g per 100g)
- Cooked fats
- Lamb, pork, mutton
- Poultry fat and beef fat
- Fizzy drinks
- Sweets
- Pastries, ices
- White bread, cereals containing chocolate or added sugars
- Cocktail snacks
- Butter
- Aperitifs (except for a small glass of wine, which is good for us).

Everything else is fine, in moderation. Don't overeat. Cut your present daily intake by half and you'll be amazed at the results. Give it a try!

## 6. Stomach Pain, Bloating, Constipation

Intestinal problems are a sign of stress, but also of poor diet which leads to formation of gas.

Listen to your body and make sure you only eat healthy foods which are good for you.

Stop eating unhealthy, problem-causing foods and choose instead a diet rich in fiber and gastric stimulants. Avoid soufflés, meringues, and fizzy drinks. Instead, go for recipes containing fennel, cucumber, cumin, lettuce, tomato, avocado, fish, certain fruits, hard-boiled eggs or green beans, which are easily digestible and prevent production of excess gas.

**And Above All:**
Eat slowly – take your time. This is fundamental!

**A Massage to Relieve Stomach Bloating:**
Lie down in a quiet place, play a little music, lock the door – cut yourself off from interruption.

Remove any clothing which constricts your midriff.

Apply a hot napkin or a hot water bottle, a good old hot water bottle like the ones our grandmothers used.

Breathe deeply, down into your stomach.

With both hands, gently massage your stomach clockwise, pressing lightly on the harder areas, between 30 and 60 rotations.

*My Special Trick:*

I drink a large beaker of tepid water every morning before breakfast. A friend of Mayotte gave me this tip. It works!

## 7. Congestion Aromatherapy Recipe

*Recipe:*

- 30 drops of eucalyptus essential oil
- 10 drops of peppermint essential oil

*Directions:*

1. Blend the essential oils together in a dark- glass bottle.
2. Put 4-5 drops on the cotton ball and bring it near your nose. Inhale occasionally.

## 8. Detox massage

We are forever planning to take proper care of ourselves, but so often, we then give up. Here's a little preparation to apply after showering, which helps drain the body and eliminate toxins. You'll be surprised how well it works and won't want to do without it. No more need for expensive creams which, as often as not, don't work anyway.

You can make this draining preparation yourself.

*Recipe:*

- 30 cl of grape seed oil
- 10 drops of essential oil of geranium. This essential oil is a tonic and combats nervous stress.
- It disinfects the intestine and is an excellent dewormer
- 10 drops of essential oil of rosemary. This is excellent for drainage of liver and pancreas, as well as being anti-infection and anti-bacterial

- 10 drops of essential oil of lemon grass. This is a tonic which stimulates and decongests veins
- 10 drops of cypress. Essential oil of cypress helps eliminate cellulite and fat as well as improving drainage

## *Directions:*

1. Mix well.
2. Start with the left arm, work towards the chest, and then finish with the right arm.
3. Massage the legs firmly, starting from the soles of the feet and working up towards the groin.

You will experience a feeling of wellbeing such as you have never felt before. Breathe deeply and lie down to maximize the draining effect of this treatment.

I do this daily; my skin has become supple, my body firmer and each time I enjoy the wonderful feeling of freshness and lightness.
Store this preparation in a cool, dark place.

# 3 - Healthy Essential Oil Recipes For Weight Loss

## 9. DIY Weight Loss Recipes

There are countless essential oil recipes for weight loss. This chapter lists some of the most widely used recipes that, when accompanied with a healthy lifestyle, will enable you to reach your weight loss goals.

Keep in mind that essential oils are dense and highly concentrated. If you plan on applying essential oils topically, avoid doing so in their undiluted form. Dilute the essential oil first with a carrier oil of your choice to make the oil mild enough for topical application.

This blend takes four key essential oils and combines their powerful effects into one effective oil blend for shedding body fat. If your budget doesn't allow for a visit to an aromatherapist, this blend is a relatively inexpensive alternative—and incredibly easy to make, too.

## *Recipe:*

- 5 drops of peppermint essential oil
- 10 drops of bergamot essential oil
- 10 drops of sandalwood essential oil
- 15 drops of grapefruit essential oil
- A ceramic bowl
- A clean spoon
- A dark tinted glass vial
- Carrier oil as needed

## *Directions:*

1. Start by combining all of the essential oils in a clean bowl, and mix well.
2. Carefully pour the blend into a vial. Shake well.

3. Use ten drops of the blend for every bath, making sure to soak for at least 30 minutes while massaging the areas of your body where fat tends to accumulate.
4. For a quick massage, simply dilute 1-2 drops of the essential oil blend in an ounce of almond, jojoba, coconut, or extra virgin olive oil. Massage the mixture into your cellulite-prone areas, your forehead, the back of your neck, or your feet.
5. This special blend also works great in your diffuser. 6-8 drops should do the trick.

## 10. Weight Loss Shot

The last thing you need if you're trying to shed a few unwanted pounds is alcohol. However, this recipe allows you to take shots without harming your health. It includes absolutely zero alcohol— just the slimming and therapeutic benefits of three essential oils. This shot improves metabolism and digestion, significantly reduces stress and wards off midday and midnight cravings. It offers approximately one week of use, so feel free to double or triple the ingredients for prolonged usage.

### Recipe:

- 5 drops of either grapefruit or lemon essential oil
- 5 drops of bergamot essential oil
- 5 drops of frankincense essential oil
- A tinted glass vial with dropper

### Directions:

1. Add all three essential oils in a vial and shake to combine.
2. Fill a shot glass with water or fresh orange juice. Add 1-2 drops of the oil blend. Bottoms up!
3. Repeat three times a day before each meal, or anytime stress or cravings raise their ugly heads.

## 11. Slimming Beverage

This recipe combines five weight-reducing essential oils for the ultimate weight loss drink. It works great as an appetite suppressant and is mild enough to drink throughout the day. In fact, it is recommended to drink this beverage as often as four times a day as essential oils are quickly absorbed and utilized by your body.

Supplying your body with a consistent flow of essential oils is important for ultimate efficacy. This beverage also promotes sleep: proper rest is a key tool for any weight loss plan.

### *Recipe:*

- 20 drops of cinnamon essential oil (Make sure to use essential oil derived from cinnamon bark.)
- 40 drops of grapefruit essential oil
- 40 drops of lemon essential oil
- 40 drops of ginger essential oil
- 40 drops of peppermint essential oil
- A 15ml tinted glass vial with dropper

### *Directions:*

1. Put all of the essential oils into a vial and shake to combine well. Your vial should be nearly full once you've added all of the ingredients.
2. Before each meal, dilute two drops of the oil blend in a glass cup of cool mineral water, and drink.

## 12. Weight problems

You are overweight.

Do you want to get rid of those unsightly bulges?

Cypress is effective against fat deposits and cellulite. It is also excellent for vascular drainage. Lemon grass is a tonic which stimulates and decongests veins. Juniper promotes active metabolism. Mint refreshes and stimulates circulation

## *Recipe:*

After showering, massage with the following preparation:

- 100 ml of avocado oil
- 20 drops of essential oil of cypress
- 20 drops of essential oil of lemon grass
- 20 drops of essential oil of juniper
- 10 drops of essential oil of mint.

## *Directions:*

1. Place a few drops of cypress in your ear overnight. This will promote weight loss. Above all, during your diet, choose foods which are light, rich in fiber and contain little fat and sugar. Cut your daily intake by half, keep moving, walk upstairs instead of taking the lift, skip around, and be active.

Take good care of yourself. You are an important person and nothing should trouble you.

# 4 - Healthy Essential Oil Recipes for Bath Time

### 13. Relaxing Bath-Time

No stress. Learn how to relax and to forget job-related pressure. Breath in, breath out! Relax, take care of yourself, and you will feel, day by day, ever lighter and more serene.

Here is how to have a relaxing bath which will increase your feelings of sensuality and serenity:

*Recipe:*

- 2 spoon full of whole milk, in a glass
- 4 drops of essential oil of rosemary
- 4 drops of essential oil of sandalwood
- 2 drops of essential oil of rose
- 2 drops of essential oil of sage

Add to the bathwater just before getting in. Let yourself go...

### 14. Stimulating Bath-Time

Make up the following bath foam, before an evening out after work:

*Recipe:*

- Mix 25 ml of glycerin (available at your local chemist) with 120ml of unperfumed liquid soap
- Add 35 drops of essential oil of lemon grass. This is a stimulating tonic
- 15 drops of essential oil of ginger. This essential oil combats fatigue and is a stimulant
- 15 drops of angelica. This is an invigorating essential oil which combats sexual fatigue

- Stir vigorously
- Pour 2 soup-spoons full under the running tap to dissolve it into your bathwater

You can prepare large amounts of this bath foam, as long as you have a cool, dark place to store it.

## 15. Relaxing Lavender Oil

Relaxing lavender oil after a stressful day. Lavender is a tonic for the veins, an analgesic for headaches and also has relaxing properties.

## *Recipe:*

*Mix*

- 10 cl of grape seed oil
- 5 drops of essential oil of Lavandula Officinalis

Apply to the nape of the neck, the forehead, the temples or the upper back.

## *In the Bath:*
Mix 5 drops in a little bath foam.
A few drops on a handkerchief, inhale.

*Lavender has numerous beneficial properties:* inter alia, it soothes and regulates the nervous system. It slightly lowers arterial pressure, it improves circulation, is antiseptic and calms insect bites.

# 5 - Healthy Essential Oils Recipe for Injury

## 16. Minor Cuts Aromatherapy Salve Recipe

If you would prefer an alternative to antibiotic ointments that contain chemicals and no petroleum jelly, you'll love this. Use sweet almond oil as your carrier oil.

Apply a small amount of the balm to the cut or scrape and then apply a bandage if necessary.

### Recipe:

- 3 oz. of carrier oil.
- 1 oz. beeswax that's been grated
- 40 drops of tea tree essential oil
- 40 drops of lavender essential oil

### Directions:

1. Place the beeswax in a double boiler and heat on low. In a separate pan, slowly heat your carrier oil.
2. Pour the warm carrier oil into a bowl, and add the melted beeswax.
3. Stir very well.
4. Add the lavender and tea tree essential oils and continue to stir.
5. Pour the mixture into a glass jar. Let cool and then place the lid on the jar.

## 17. Bruising Aromatherapy Recipe

Helichyrysum essential oil has significant anti-inflammatory qualities. It will ease discomfort and reduce bruising coloring.

**Blend #1**

- 1 oz. sweet almond oil
- 8 drops of roman chamomile essential oil

## Blend #2

- 1 oz. jojoba
- 8 drops of Helichrysum essential oil

## Blend #3

- 1 oz. sweet almond oil or jojoba
- 8 drops of yarrow essential oil

## *Directions:*

1. Mix the essential oils with the carrier oil.
2. Store in a dark glass bottle.

# 6 - Healthy Essential Oil Recipes For Lifestyle

### 18. Essential oil Aromatherapy Recipes

Massage is a valuable tool to reduce stress and relax the body.

## *Recipe:*

- 4 fl ounces of sweet almond oil
- 30 drops of essential oil. Choose oils that will compliment your massage and that are safe to apply to the skin.

## Sleep Inducing Blend

- 30 drops roman chamomile

## Aphrodisiac Blend

- 10 drops jasmine essential oil
- 20 drops sandalwood essential oil

## Stress Blend

- 10 drops lavender essential oil
- 5 drops lemon essential oil
- 15 drops Clary sage essential oil

## Sore Muscle Blend

- 4 drops black pepper essential oil
- 6 drops ginger essential oil
- 10 drops peppermint essential oil
- 10 drops eucalyptus essential oil

## *Directions:*

1. Mix the oils together and store in a dark glass container. You can double the recipe if you like.
2. Apply a small amount for massaging.

*Disclaimer:* Make sure that you know how to safely give a massage.

## 19. Blends to Calm and Relax

These recipes can help to calm and relax.

### Blend #1

- 3 drops frankincense essential oil
- 2 drops lavender essential oil
- 1 drop Roman chamomile essential oil

### Blend #2

- 4 drops lavender essential oil
- 2 drops Roman chamomile essential oil

### Blend #3

- 4 drops lavender essential oil
- 2 drops Roman chamomile essential oil
- 1 drop frankincense essential oil

## 20. Deep Hair Conditioner Recipe

*Recipe:*

- 4 tablespoon jojoba
- 10 drops rosemary essential oil
- 3 drops lavender essential oil

*Directions:*

1. The recipe makes one dose. You can make larger quantities and store in a glass bottle if you want.
2. Mix the Jojoba and rosemary essential oil in a small bowl.
3. Use warm water to wet your hair.
4. Apply the conditioning blend.
5. Leave on your hair for 60 minutes. Wash as normal.

Jojoba and rosemary are moisturizing to your hair and rosemary helps control dandruff.

## 21. Menstrual Cramp Recipe

Menstrual cramps can be very painful and they can interfere with your day-to-day activities. Gently massage into your abdomen to reduce cramps and pain.

### Ingredients:

- 2 oz sweet almond oil
- 16 drops peppermint essential oil
- 6 drops lavender essential oil
- 2 drops cypress essential oil

### Directions:

1. Mix the essential oils and almond oil together in a dark-colored glass bottle. Rotate from side to side to mix.
2. Gently massage a small amount into the abdominal area.

## 22. Insect Repellent Recipe

If you love spending time outdoors, but you hate being bit and you hate toxic chemical insect repellents just as much as bug bites, then this is for you.

This insect repellent smells nice and contains no toxic ingredients. It's quite effective at keeping insects at bay. Do a skin test before you use and remember its effectiveness is linked to your body chemistry.

## Recipe:

- 3 oz. of high-proof alcohol - vodka works great.
- 40 drops of citronella essential oil
- 15 drops of eucalyptus essential oil
- 15 drops of lemongrass essential oil
- 10 drops of lavender essential oil

## Directions:

1. Fill your glass bottle with the alcohol and essential oils. If you have a glass spritzer bottle, that's perfect.
2. Shake well each time before you use it to ensure the oils are mixed in the alcohol, and then mist your skin and clothing. Reapply as needed.

# 7 - Healthy Essential Oil Recipes For Sanitation

### 23. General Sanitation Essential Oil Recipe

You probably have found yourself buying different commercial toilet cleaners after watching them being advertised on your television. Yes, some of these products will leave your toilet sparkling clean, but they also contain toxic chemicals that put your family's health at risk if used in the long term. That is why it is better to formulate your own cleaner, using natural ingredients that are safe for your family. Here's how to make a natural toilet cleaner with essential oils.

*Recipe:*

- A cup of distilled white vinegar
- 1 cup of baking soda
- 15 drops of tea tree oil

*Directions:*

1. Mix the vinegar and the tea tree oil in a spray bottle and shake well.
2. Spray the mixture in your toilet bowl, as well as on the lid, seat, and handle.
3. Wait for the mixture to settle for at least 30 minutes, sprinkle the baking soda inside the bowl, scrub with a toilet brush, and flush.
4. Using a clean and dry towel, wipe the vinegar solution from the seat, lid, and handle.

This deodorizing formula uses tea tree oil's antibacterial properties to kill germs in the toilet.

Alternatively, you can also use the below recipe if you have stubborn stains that refuse to away even after using regular toilet cleaners.

## *Recipe:*

- 1 cup of borax
- 1 cup of white vinegar
- 5 drops of lemon essential oil
- 10 drops of lavender essential oil

## *Directions*:

1. Mix all the ingredients in a bottle.
2. Flush the toilet to wet it.
3. Pour the mixture into your toilet bowl, and let it sit for several hours. If you can, allow it to sit overnight, ensuring that none of your family members use the toilet during the time.
4. Scrub the bowl thoroughly, and then flush the toilet to rinse.

It's worth noting that borax is not similar to boric acid, which is toxic. On the contrary, it is sodium tetraborate, which is a multi-purpose cleaner that deodorizes, whitens and removes stains.

Just like baking soda, or table salt, borax can only be poisonous when used in very large amounts.

Borax and white vinegar are natural cleaning agents that help to disinfect and remove stains. On the other hand, lavender and lemon oils have anti-microbial and deodorizing properties, which help to kill germs and eliminating stale odors. Together, they'll leave your toilet extremely clean, and smelling nice too.

## 24. Natural Toothpaste

Why continue spending money to buy toothpaste when you can make your own at home using all natural ingredients? And the best part, it takes less than five minutes to prepare. Here's how:

## *Recipe:*

- 10 drops of peppermint essential oil (use your favorite flavor)
- 1 tablespoon of fine sea salt (the minerals in the sea salt are great for your teeth, but you can leave it out if you find the taste too salty for you)
- 2/3 cup of baking soda
- Filtered water

## *Directions:*

1. Mix together the baking soda, peppermint oil, and sea salt.
2. Add a small amount of water at a time, and stir after each addition, till the paste reaches your desired co
3. That's it. No more excuses for having bad breath or stained teeth.

The above ingredients can make an equivalent of a 5.3 oz. tube full of toothpaste, so it will take a while before you make another one. To use, just wet your toothbrush, spread the toothpaste on the brush, and begin brushing. When not in use, store the preparation in a cool, dry place, preferably next to your toothbrush.

## Heartburn Essential Oil Blend

## *Ingredients:*
- 1 drop of peppermint essential oil
- 2 drops of eucalyptus essential oil
- 2 drops of fennel oil
- 1 tsp of grape seed oil

## *Directions:*

Mix these oils and use the blend to rub the upper abdominal area.

## 25. Essential Oil Mouthwash for Fighting Gingivitis

*Recipe:*

- 1 tbsp of brandy
- 3 drops of peppermint essential oil
- 3 drops of thyme essential oil
- 3 drops of chamomile essential oil
- 2 drops of eucalyptus essential oil

*Directions:*

1. Mix the oils and dissolve one tsp of the mixture in a glass of warm water.
2. Swish the warm water and oil mixture in your mouth but do not swallow.

## 26. Essential Oil Mouthwash for Bad Breathe

*Recipe:*

- 2 drops of tea tree oil
- 2 drops of geranium oil
- 2 drops of thyme oil
- 2 drops of lemon oil
- 2 drops of peppermint oil
- 10 ml brandy

*Directions:*

Mix all the oils and dissolve a teaspoon in a glass of water, swish around your mouth then spit out.

## 27. Essential Oil Mouthwash to Help with Bleeding Gums

### *Recipe:*

- 3 drops of peppermint oil
- 3 drops of thyme
- 3 drops of chamomile oil
- 2 drops of eucalyptus oil
- 1 tbsp of brandy

### *Directions:*

1. Mix these oils and dissolve in one tablespoon of brandy.
2. Use a teaspoon of the oils in a glass of warm water.
3. Swish the warm water with the mixture around your mouth, then spit; do not swallow.

# 8 - Healthy Essential Oil Recipes for Allergy

### 28. Natural Sinus Infection Treatment

If you've had a sinus infection before, then you know how awful it feels. The constant headaches, the stuffy nose, and loss of smell are symptoms that no one loves to go through. Fortunately, there are natural remedies that can help cure the infection for good. Essential oils, such as eucalyptus or peppermint oil, have anti-microbial properties, which makes them a powerful tool for treating sinus infections.

*Recipe:*

- 1 drop of peppermint or eucalyptus oil
- 1 tablespoon of coconut oil

*Directions:*

Dilute the peppermint or eucalyptus oil in the carrier oil (coconut), and apply to the bridge of your nose. These essential oils are natural humidifiers, which help to open up nasal passages.

Alternatively, you can also use frankincense to clear up the stuffiness. Take advantage of the above simple, essential oil recipes, to make effective homemade products that are cheap and safe to use.

### 29. Allergy Relief Cream

*Recipe:*

Essential Oils:
- 10 drops of Peppermint
- 10 drops of Lavender
- 10 drops of Lemon
- 1/4 coconut oil (whipped for 5 minutes)

## Directions:

Compared to other essential oil concoctions, this product is a thicker topical blend that is so easy to prepare. All you have to do is to mix all the ingredients thoroughly then store in a glass jar. Apply on the affected areas to soothe allergy effects.

## 30. DIY Hay Fever Inhaler I

## Recipe:

Essential Oils:
- 3 drops of Roman Chamomile
- 3 drops of German Chamomile
- 2 drops of Helichrysum
- 2 drops of Lavender
- 1 drop of Peppermint (optional)
- 1 clean, empty personal inhaler bottle

## Directions:

Blend all essential oils then pour into the refillable inhaler. When hay fever symptoms become apparent, inhale this blend into each nostril once. Do this every six to eight hours to stop frequent sneezing and watery eyes.

## 31. DIY Hay Fever Inhaler II

## Recipe:

Essential Oils:
- 8 drops of German Chamomile
- 4 drops of Helichrysum
- 4 drops of Geranium

- 3 drop of Eucalyptus
- 3 drops of Rosemary
- 1 clean, empty personal inhaler bottle

## Directions:

Blend all essential oils in the refillable inhaler. When hay fever symptoms become apparent, inhale this blend into each nostril once. Do this every six to eight hours to prevent frequent sneezing and watery eyes.

Note: German chamomile is a known natural antihistamine that deters sneezing.

## 32. Essential Oil Blend Concentrate for Hay Fever

## Recipe:

Essential Oils:
- 3 drops of Tea Tree
- 3 drops of Sandalwood
- 2 drops of Rosemary
- 1 oz. carrier oil (ex. Sunflower oil, jojoba oil)

## Directions:

Mix all essential oils together then add into an ounce of carrier oil. You can use this mixture for massaging the chest and face to relieve nasal congestion.

## 33. General Allergy Relief

## Recipe:

Essential Oils:
- 3 drops of Lavender
- 3 drops of Lemon

- 3 drops of Peppermint
- 1 tablespoon of honey

## *Directions:*

Add the lavender, lemon, and peppermint essential oils to a spoonful of honey. Mix well. You can apply this directly on inflamed parts of the skin or take orally.

## 34. Nasal Allergy Spray

## *Recipe:*

Essential Oils:
- 4 drops of Frankincense
- 6 drops of Lavender
- Distilled water
- A pinch of fine Himalayan salt

## *Directions:*

Mix frankincense, lavender and Himalayan salt in a nose spray bottle. Fill in the rest of the bottle with distilled water then shake well. Store it in a cool, dry place. Use as needed. If you are using Himalayan salt crystals, remember to crush it first using a mortar and pestle before blending with the oils.

## 35. Natural Blend for Respiratory Allergies

## *Recipe:*

Essential Oils:
- 2 drops of Basil
- 2 drops of Rosemary
- 2 drops of Lemon

- 2 drops of Orange
- 1 drop of Tea tree
- 1 drop of Thyme
- 1 drop of Ginger

## *Directions:*

1. This blend is perfect for diffusing in your bedroom or family room to help your loved ones experience some relief from any allergic attack.
2. Just mix all of the essential oils in a dropper bottle.
3. Then, add about three to five drops of the blend to a diffuser.
4. Enjoy the wonderful, refreshing scents!

## 36. Decongesting Allergy Bomb I

## *Recipe:*

Essential Oils:
- 2 drops of Lemon
- 2 drops of Lavender
- 2 drops of Peppermint
- 2 drops of Melaleuca
- Vegetable capsule

## *Directions:*

1. Mix in all essentials oils in a veggie capsule.
2. When an allergic reaction strikes, take one capsule for immediate relief.

## 37. Decongesting Allergy Bomb II (*strengthened*)

## *Recipe:*

Essential Oils:
- 5 drops of Lemon
- 5 drops of Lavender
- 5 drops of Peppermint
- 3 drops of Copaiba
- Vegetable capsule

## *Directions:*

1. Combine in a capsule lemon, lavender and peppermint oils.
2. Seal well and store in a clean, dry container.

Take one capsule for immediate relief when sinus congestion starts. For added strength, just add three drops of copaiba.

# 9 - Essential Oil Recipes for Colds and Flu

### 38. Essential Oil Recipe for Flu, Colds and Coughs

*Recipe:*

- 2 drops of eucalyptus essential oil
- 2 drops of lavender essential oil
- 2 drops of tea tree essential oil

*Directions:*

1. Boil a pot of water and remove from the heat source.
2. While steaming, add in the eucalyptus, lavender and tea tree essential oils.
3. Cover your head with a towel as you inhale the steam for at least three minutes. Always ensure that your eyes are closed.

### 39. Recipe For Eeasing Coughs

*Recipe:*

- 2 drops of lavender essential oil
- 2 drops of eucalyptus essential oil

*Directions:*

Boil a pot of water and remove from the heat. As it is still steaming, add the eucalyptus and lavender oils. Immediately, cover the pot and your head with a towel and inhale the steam for around three minutes while your eyes are closed. If you would want to ease the coughing throughout the day, it is advisable to add the eucalyptus oil and lavender to a carrier oil and apply on your chest and throat.

## 40. Essential Oil to Reduce Fever

*Recipe:*

- 1 drop of tea tree essential oil
- 1 drop of rosemary essential oil
- 2 drops of peppermint essential oil
- 1 drop of black pepper essential oil
- 2 drops eucalyptus essential oil
- 2 drops of lavender essential oil
- 15 ml of evening primrose oil

*Directions:*

Mix the oils and massage your temples, soles of feet, tops of hands and the back of your neck.

## 41. Essential Oil Blend to Help With Difficulty in Breathing

*Recipe:*

- 3 drops of rosemary oil
- 10 drops of eucalyptus oil
- 10 drops of ginger oil
- 5 drops of nutmeg oil
- 2 drops of cinnamon oil
- 30 ml of vegetable carrier oil

*Directions:*
This Essential oil mixture needs to be rubbed around the back and chest.

# Conclusion

Thank you again for purchasing this book!

The recipes contained in this guide are designed to be made up by
anyone, without any specialized knowledge. Please just bear in mind
the warnings mentioned at the beginning of the guide.
Nothing should stand between you and your wellbeing. You are
unique and precious and you ought to take care of yourself.

I hope you will find enjoy this guide and that you will give your body
the care it deserves.

Did you find these suggestions and recipes useful? If you enjoyed this
book tell your friends and spread the world.

Thank you and good luck! – Kathy Lewis

## ABOUT THE AUTHOR

Kathy Lewis is a Dermatologist whose interest in using natural supplements to heal skin. While helping others at the office she loves to travel with her husband once a month to different countries. Exploring almost 13 so far. Kathy also loves to write while on her free time, especially about Essential Oils.

www.ingramcontent.com/pod-product-compliance
Lightning Source LLC
Chambersburg PA
CBHW071259280526
45788CB00004B/1782

* 9 7 8 1 5 2 2 9 9 7 7 4 0 *